Anesthesia and women's common diseases

HALA MOSTAFA GOMA
Professor of Anesthesia Cairo University

Table of contents

Introduction

Women may be subjected to anesthesia much time across her life.as women as regards certain diseases may be higher than men, on the other hand ,certain obstetric diseases concerned women only. Many factors control women and anesthesia, as the physiological difference between women and men, the higher prevalence of certain diseases and the age of women. The top diseases of women are heart diseases, cancer, autoimmune diseases, osteoporosis, and depression. In this book I will focus on risk factors for each disease and the anesthetic consideration of it.

Physiological difference between women and men
Factors affecting physiological differences between women and men:
- Sex-linked genetic illnesses
- Parts of the reproductive system that are specific to one sex
- Social causes that relate to the gender role expected of that sex in a particular society.
- Different levels of prevention, reporting, diagnosis or treatment in each gender.

Women and cardiac diseases
Anatomic differences:

- The size of the heart and major blood vessels of women are smaller than those of men of the same race and age
- The anatomic location of the major vessels in the heart, lung, and most organs are indistinguishable among the sexes.
- The cardiovascular systems of males and females have the same formed elements circulating in the blood,
- The vessels are composed of the same cell types, and the union of the elements performs the same functions.
- Healthy men and women are nearly the same.

- Men respond to psychological stress with higher increases in cortisol, compared to women.
- This greater activation of the Hypothalamus-Pituitary axis could translate into an elevated risk for CVD, diabetes and hypertension and may be linked to the higher prevalence of these diseases in men.
- Gender differences in brain structures and/or cognitive processes may be responsible for these sexually dimorphic stress responses

- men are at greater risk, and their incidence of hypertension is greater than for premenopausal women of the same age .
- men have higher blood pressures than premenopausal,
- After menopause, the sex difference in the incidence of hypertension is lost
- there is significant evidence for a role for both testosterone in the development of and estrogen in the protection against high blood pressure.

Neurohumoral control cardiovascular system.
The aim neurohumoral mechanisms are to ensure the cardiac, cerebral and renal optimal function.
- sympatho vagal balance
- Vagal and sympathetic systems and by their interaction,
- Fertile women show a predominant vagal tone.
- An increased sympathetic tone is found in
- Arterial hypertension,
- Diabetes,
- Chronic heart failure
- Myocardial infarction.

Hormonal control of the cardiovascular system
- Renin-angiotensin
- catecholamine,
- insulin

- Estrogens,
- Men had greater cortisol and diastolic blood pressure responses compared to women.

Risk factors you can be controlled include:
- High blood cholesterol and triglyceride levels (a type of fat found in the blood)
- High blood pressure.
- Diabetes and prediabetes.
- Overweight and obesity.
- Smoking.
- Lack of physical activity.
- Unhealthy diet.
- Stress

Cardiac diseases, risk factors for women are

- smoking,
- use of oral contraceptives,
- diabetes,
- elevated blood pressure,
- elevated blood lipids,
- low socio-economic status,
- low educational attainment,
- Type A behavior and chronic troubling emotions
- Estrogen replacement therapy seems to protect against coronary heart disease, although the reduction in risk may have been over-estimated.

- Elevated cholesterol and elevated blood pressure are major risk factors, and diabetes seems to have a stronger impact on risk in women than in men. Low
- Socio-economic class is a stronger risk factor for women than for men and the double loads of career and family seem to increase risk for women.

The social and psychological risks for CHD:
- Behavior patterns of individuals (eg. type A personality)
- Hostility.
- Social support.
- Hopelessness.
- Depression.
- Social class.
- Education.

High risk patients for perioperative cardiac complications
- Significant coronary artery disease
- left ventricular systolic dysfunction (left ventricular ejection fraction ≤ 40 percent)

- cerebrovascular disease
- peripheral artery disease compared with matched controls
- Physiologic factors associated with surgery predisposed to myocardial
- Ischemia, which is more pronounced in patients with underlying coronary disease.

- **Intraoperative risk factors**

- Volume shifts and blood loss,
- Enhanced myocardial oxygen demand from elevations in heart rate and blood pressure secondary to stress from surgery,
- Increase in postoperative platelet reactivity

peioperative cardiac complications are
- MI.
- HF.
- ventricular fibrillation.
- primary cardiac arrest.
- complete heart block.
- cardiac death.

Very high-risk patients
- recent myocardial infarction (MI)
- unstable angina,
- decompensated heart failure (HF),

- high-grade arrhythmias,
- hemodynamically important valvular heart disease (aortic stenosis in particular) All such patients should be optimally treated, with possible referral to a cardiologist for further evaluation and management.

Anesthesia and ischemic patients

- Surgical stress induces:
- Autonomic, sympathetic stimulation which increases myocardial oxygen demand by both positive chronoscopic (increased heart rate) and positive inotropic (increased contractility)
- Increased circulating catecholamine and direct cardiac stimulation by norepinephrine release from sympathetic ending
- Increased BP increases oxygen demand and coronary blood flow; decreased BP may promote reduced coronary flow

Goal for anesthesia:

- Prevention/treatment of Intraoperative cardiac ischemia -- method:
- Minimize cardiac O2 demand

- Maximize cardiac O2 supply

<u>Factors controlling the Myocardial Oxygen Supply:</u>

Auto regulation: Constant flow despite significant blood-pressure variations
Anemia: blood flow increases to ensure adequate O2 delivery to the myocardium
- With maximal vasodilatation, coronary blood flow is related linearly to blood pressure

<u>Factors increase Myocardial Oxygen Demand:</u>
- Increased Myocardial wall tension
- Increased Cardiac contractility

<u>Intraoperative measures for prevention of excessive myocardial O2 demand</u>:
- Excessive myocardial contractility may be reduced by anesthetics, which act by limiting sympathetic stimulation

- With adequate cardiac function ß-adrenoceptor blocking agents may be used to diminish contractility

Effects of anemia:
- Anemia increases myocardial O2 demand while concurrently reducing myocardial O2 supply
- Correction of intraoperative blood loss by blood transfusion.

Balancing myocardial O2 supply and O2 demand requirements

1: ß-adrenoceptor blockade (e.g., propranolol (Inderal); metoprolol (Lopressor)
- Reduces cardiac O2 demand by attenuating contractility (negative inotropism) increases mediated by increased circulating catecholamine levels and sympathetic nervous system activity

- Reduced heart rate (negative chronotropism) increases diastolic filling time, thereby increasing time available for coronary vascular perfusion
- It reduced myocardial oxygen consumption (reduced afterload)
- reduced coronary blood flow through stenotic regions
- both limitation in myocardial oxygen demand and maximization of supply: anesthetic should optimize this balance

Maintenance of diastolic blood pressure:
- A significant percentage of epicardial and nearly all middle cardial and endocardial coronary flow occurs during diastole
- Tachycardia: decreases diastolic interval and reduce coronary flow
- avoiding conditions producing tachycardia
- bradycardia is not desirable in terms of increasing epicardial coronary flow
- In patients with coronary vascular disease, the pressure gradient which drives coronary blood flow may be small in influence significantly by LVEDP (wedge pressure)

Anesthetic measures:

Properly chosen anesthetic agents block the stress response; β-adrenergic receptor blockers also only used to avoid increased contractility/rate.

- Improve oxygenation
- Adequate tidal volume
- Positive end expiratory pressure (PEEP)
- Insure high inspired oxygen
- Treat anemia with blood transfusion

3 .**Monitor ventricular filling pressures** using the pulmonary artery catheter
Nitroglycerin may be used to maintain optimal filling pressure
4. Optimization of coronary perfusion pressure gradients involved typically:
- Raising the diastolic arterial pressure
- Decreasing LVEDP (left ventricular and diastolic pressure)
- With left ventricular heart failure, inotropic support may improve the relationship between oxygen supply and demand

5. Optimize coronary flow by maintaining blood-pressure at or slightly above normal (may require α-adrenoceptor agonist administration.
6. Prevent increased heart rate using anesthetic agents initially and β-receptor blockade as needed.
7. Increased ventricular filling pressures reduce coronary blood flow, particularly subendocardial flow. Maintain reduced filling pressures using nitroglycern
8. Provide optimal oxygenation.

Autoimmune diseases, and Women

- Autoimmune diseases affect women three times more than men.
- Since the women affected are mostly young women in their childbearing years, a time when they are traditionally most healthy, getting a diagnosis can prove to be extremely difficult.
- Some diseases have an even higher incidence in women. Autoimmune diseases have been cited in the top ten leading causes of all deaths in women age 65 and younger.
- Male-predominant autoimmune diseases usually manifest clinically (ie, show signs and symptoms of clinical disease) before age 50 and are characterized by acute inflammation and a Th1-type response, whereas autoimmune diseases with an increased

incidence in females that occur early in life have a clear antibody-mediated pathology.

- Autoimmune diseases with an increased incidence in females appear clinically later in life when chronic pathology, fibrosis, and increased numbers of autoantibodies are present. This distinction between acute and chronic pathology in autoimmune diseases,
- The number of different autoantibodies present in an individual is a good predictor of the risk of developing an autoimmune disease.

Possible causes of the high incidence of autoimmune diseases in women than men

- women have enhanced immune systems compared to men increases women's resistance to many types of infection
- They are more susceptible to ADs.
- Women who have an autoimmune disease have suffered from a lack of focus and a scattered research approach.

- autoimmunity is known to have a genetic basis and tends to cluster in families as different autoimmune diseases
- Different ethnic groups are more susceptible to certain autoimmune diseases.
- Women respond to infection, vaccination, and trauma with increased antibody production, whereas

inflammation is usually more severe in men resulting in an increased mortality in men and protection against infection in women

- Women respond to infection, vaccination, and trauma with increased antibody production, whereas inflammation is usually more severe in men resulting in an increased mortality in men and protection against infection in women
- Antibodies provide critical protection against infection, and are the key protective response induced by vaccination.
- autoantibodies may induce damage by binding self-antigens and activating the complement cascade, resulting in direct cytotoxicity or an immune complex (IC)-associated pathology

Female: Male Ratios in Autoimmune Diseases	
Hashimoto's thyroiditis	10:1
Systemic lupus erythematous	9:1
Sjogren's syndrome	9:1
Ant phospholipid syndrome-secondary	9:1
Primary biliary cirrhosis	9:1
Autoimmune hepatitis	8:1
Graves' disease	7:1
Scleroderma	3:1
Rheumatoid arthritis	2.5:1
Antiphospholipid syndrome-primary	2:1

Autoimmune thrombocytopenic purpura (ITP)	2:1
Multiple sclerosis	2:1
Myasthenia gravis	2:1

Autoimmune Disease Diagnosis

- Symptoms vary widely, notably from one illness to another and even within the same disease. And because the diseases affect multiple body systems, their symptoms are often misleading, which hinders accurate diagnosis.
- Autoimmune diseases remain among the most poorly understood and poorly recognized of any category of illness. Individual diseases range from the benign to the severe.

Measures needed for early diagnosis of autoimmune diseases in women

1. Recognizing autoimmunity as a "category" of disease. Be more aware of the genetic predisposition to develop autoimmune disease, clearly there would be more emphasis on taking a medical history regarding autoimmune diseases within the family when presented by a patient with confusing symptoms.
2. Increasing public education about autoimmunity and autoimmune disease.
3. Creating Autoimmune Diagnostic Triage Clinics or Autoimmune Centers of Excellence. These
4. Facilitating more collaboration and cross fertilization of basic autoimmune research.

Anesthetic considerations of specific autoimmune diseases

Systemic lupus erythematosus

- It is ranging from relatively mild and uncomplicated to major life-threatening disease.
- Anesthetic management taking into account severity of the disease.
- The potential drug interactions with immunosuppressant
- An unexpected difficult airway with subglottic stenosis or laryngeal edema
- Coagulation profile of the patient.

Cardiovascular involvement
pericarditis, my**ocarditis, arthrosclerosis, and the myocardial ischemia**
Pulmonary involvement

- pleuritis, pleural effusion, alveolar hemorrhage, and interstitial lung disease
- Renal involvement is seen in the form of lupus nephritis characterized by proteinuria, hematuria, and abnormal urinary segments
- Patients with SLE are at high risk of hypertension renal status. High-dose prednisolone and developed hypertension.

Central and peripheral nervous system complications

- A 37-95% of SLE patients may manifest central and peripheral nervous system complications.
- Headaches, seizures, cerebrovascular disease, psychosis, acute confusional states to even demyelinating disease states. hemi paresis and improved by physical rehabilitation.

Hematological manifestations
- Hematological manifestations commonly seen in SLE include
- Anemia, thrombocytopenia, and leucopenia. Anemia is found in about half of SLE patients with the most common cause being anemia of chronic disease; however, other causes include autoimmune hemolytic anemia, iron deficiency anemia, anemia of chronic renal failure, and cyclophosphamide myelotoxicity.

Joints affection

- Nonerosive arthritis is seen in patients with SLE. Prolonged glucocorticoid use for immunosuppression could cause osteoporosis.
- Incidence of atlantoaxial subluxation has been reported.

Obstetric complications
Antiphospholipid syndrome may occur secondary to SLE and is characterized clinically by recurrent pregnancy loss and by presence of lupus anticoagulant antibodies which may falsely prolong activated partial thromboplastin time in such individuals

Preoperative preparation
- The preoperative aims
- he activity of the lupus
- organ damage
- medication exposure
- preanesthetic assessment, and laboratory test.
- Care of the high-risk patients requires a multidisciplinary approach.

Preoperative investigations
- Complete blood count
- coagulation profile.

- Platelet count of high risk of thrombocytopenia in lupus patients
- Electrocardiography may be done when suspecting pericarditis, myocarditis.
- chest X-ray may be reserved for extreme cases where pleural effusion or interstitial pneumonitis
- renal involvement
- creatinine clearance and 24 h urine protein
- If the patient is on steroids then, a close watch on blood glucose levels is advocated.
- Anticardiolipin antibody, lupus anticoagulant, anti-β2 glycoprotein

Intraoperative management:
  Monitoring during anesthesia includes
- Five-lead ECG, noninvasive blood pressure,
- pulse oximetry,
- Invasive monitoring should be used in patients with myocarditis, valvular involvement, or conduction abnormalities.

<u>**Renal protective strategies**</u>
- Maintenance of urine output,
- Avoidance of nephrotoxic drugs are the goals during anesthesia.
- Adequate pain management

- Corticosteroid cover should be given intraoperatively to prevent adrenal suppression.
- Antibiotics are to be given to prevent infectionPatient
- Patient should be positioned with care to avoid joint stress.

Airway management:
- Difficult airway should be anticipated in all the patients
- Smaller sized tubes and laryngeal mask airway must be available considering the potential laryngeal and the subglottic involvement.
- Laryngeal involvement could vary
- Compression of recurrent laryngeal nerve by dilated pulmonary artery has been reported as the cause of left palsy in patients with SLE.
- Secondary nerve vasculitis is believed to be a cause especially in vocal cord palsy involving right side. There is a significant risk of failed intubation and airway trauma during instrumentation.

Anesthetic drug and immunosuppressive drugs
Azathioprine, an antimetabolite immunosuppressor, may interact with muscle relaxants, and dose increases of 37% with cisatracurium, 20% with vecuronium, and 45% with pancuronium

Multiple sclerosis

- Multiple Sclerosis is an autoimmune disease of inflammation, demyelination, and axonal damage to the central nervous system .The disease progression may be subacute with relapses and remissions or chronic and progressive. Treatments include corticosteroids.
- Interferon-beta, glatiramer acetate, azathioprine, and low-dose mexthotrexate.
- Although exacerbations can be triggered by physical and emotional stress, exacerbations and remissions often occur unpredictably.

Preoperative management

- pre-operative evaluation:
- Baseline neurologic history and exam should be performed.
- Patients on corticosteroid therapy should continue therapy and may require stress dosing.

General versus regional anesthesia

- Symptoms are experienced by 20-30% of women in the post-partum period. Whether this is due to a reversal of the pregnancy-induced 'immunotolerant' state or other factors
- regional anesthesia, both spinal and epidural anesthesia has been successfully employed in parturients with multiple sclerosis

- In some studies, spinal anesthesia has been implicated in postop exacerbations whereas epidural and peripheral nerves blocks have not.
- One theory is that demyelination of the spinal cord makes it more susceptible to the neurotoxic effects of local anesthetics and the concentration of local anesthetic in the white matter of the spinal cord is higher following a spinal compared to an epidural.

General anesthesia and MS
- General anesthesia is most often used in patients with multiple sclerosis.
- Succinylcholine judiciously as demyelination and denervation may increase the risk of succinylcholine-induced hyperkalemia in these patients.
- Nondepolarizing neuromuscular blockers are safe to use although patients with multiple sclerosis may have altered sensitivity to these drugs in the setting of baseline limb weakness.
- They may also have limited 'physiologic reserve' (neurologic and respiratory) and be less able to tolerate stressors such as a mild degree of post-operative residual muscle relaxant.

- Some multiple sclerosis patients, such as those with baseline weakness or pharyngeal dysfunction, will require extended monitoring and care postoperatively.

- As in other patients with chronic brain injury, patients with MS may be expected to have some MAC reduction and delayed emergence proportionate to the severity of their disease.

Intraoperative monitoring
Temperature and minimize increases above baseline as even slight increases in body temperature may precipitate a decline in neurologic function postoperatively.

Myasthenia Gravis

Myasthenia Gravis is an autoimmune disease that attacks post-synaptic nicotinic acetylcholine receptors at the NMJ.
- There is muscle weakness and fatigue
- Ocular, bulbar (muscles involved in speech, chewing and swallowing), respiratory, and proximal skeletal muscles.
- Symptoms seem to be worse at the end of the day or after exertion.

Classification of myasthenia
1. ocular or ocular
2. non-ocular weakness.

Preoperative evaluation
- recent course of the disease
- muscle groups affected
- drug therapy
- Coexisting diseases.
- Neurology consult.

Intraoperative management

These patients can pose a challenge during anesthesia not only because of their disease process but also from the medications used to treat them (acetylcholinesterase inhibitors, steroids, etc.).

Patients with MG are resistant to succinylcholine and are exquisitely sensitive to non-depolarizing NMBs.

Diseases associated with MG include DM, thyroid disorders, SLE and RA.

Effect of morning dose of acetylcholinesterase inhibitor

- Altered patient drug requirements following surgery
- Increased vagal reflexes
- Possibility of disrupting bowel anastomoses secondary to hyperperistalsis
- Significant side effects including salivation, miosis, bradycardia and even cholinergic crisis if given NMB reversal

Risk of aspiration

- Patients with involvement of respiratory or bulbar muscles tend to have a higher risk for aspiration

- Pretreatment with metoclopramide or H2 blockers may be helpful.
- Some patients are sensitive to respiratory depressants and premedication with opioids, BZDs, or barbiturates should be considered carefully or not at all.
- Patients might remain intubated after procedure is finished and will need to be awake prior to extubation.

Indications of post-operative ventilation support following thymectomy:
1. Disease duration > 6yrs
2. Concomitant pulmonary disease
3. Peak inspiratory pressure < -25 cmH2O
4. Vital capacity < 4 mL/kg
5. Pyridostigmine dose > 750 mg/d
6. A steroid listed on a patient's medication profile indicates a higher risk and elective procedures should be postponed if possible.
7. Of note, IV pyridostigmine is 1/30 of the PO dose.
8. IVIG or plasma exchange can be used in emergent cases.

Idiopathic thrombocytopenic purpura (ITP)
- incidence of ITP is 5% among pregnant patients
- Severe thrombocytopenia (platelet count <50,000/mm 3).
- There are auto anti bodies against the platelet membrane glycoprotein. Exacerbation of

thrombocytopenia is known to occur in pregnancy and peripartum hemorrhage is very common in these patients.

- Fetal and neonatal thrombocytopenia and intraventricular bleed are possibilities but not very common.
- **Intraoperative management**
  severe thrombocytopenia in ITP requires platelet transfusion before surgery.
- IV immunoglobulin 1 g/kg reduce platelet destruction
- Perioperative methylprednisolone 1 g along with pre-operative 8 RDP transfusions covered the perioperative period.
- Each unit of RDP is assumed to increase the platelet count by 3000–5000 units/mm 3.
- Thromboelastography can help us in this scenario, but it was not available with us. Tranexamic acid, an antifibrinolytic, helps to reduce operative blood loss and blood transfusions
- Non-steroidal anti-inflammatory drugs (NSAIDs) including paracetamol were avoided.
- No intramuscular injections were given.

Anesthetic considerations of pregnant patient with severe thrombocytopenia
- General anesthesia is preferred.
- platelet transfusion preferably single donor to prevent allo-immunisation,

- IV immunoglobulins or steroids to reduce platelet destruction, maternal
- fetal/neonatal monitoring for haemorrhagic complications,
- avoid NSAIDs or other platelet lowering drugs
- Avoidance of airway trauma, nasal intubations and intramuscular injections.
- The maternal and fetal outcomes are good with appropriate management.

Rheumatoid arthritis :

RA is a systemic disease, affecting the skeletal system as well as the cardiac and pulmonary systems and often leading to a vasculitis.
Incidence:
Rheumatoid arthritis (RA) affects ~ 1% of adults.
Importantly, Patients on DMDs are at increased risk for infection
Diagnosis
Clinical and notable for morning stiffness and metacarpophalangeal involvement
Laboratory investigations
- Rheumatoid factor is elevated in 90% of patients. CRP and ESR are elevated.
- lateral radiograph of the neck. With the neck flexed, the separation of the anterior margin of the odontoid process from the posterior margin of the anterior arch of the atlas can exceed 3 mm.

Treatment:

- Commonly used disease-modifying drugs (DMDs) include methotrexate, hydroxychloroquine, sulfasalazine, infliximab (Remicade), etanercept (Enbrel), and leflunomide (Arava, inhibits dihydroorotate dehydrogenase which is involved in pyrimidine synthesis).
- Patients may also be on NSAIDs and/or glucocorticoids
- These drugs increase risk of infection.

Intraoperative management

Airway management:
- limited mandibular motion
- mouth opening
- a narrowed glottis
- Cervical instability (subluxation, which is caused by ligamentous laxity, is present in almost 50%).
- atlantoaxial subluxation
- Consequent separation of the atlanto-odontoid articulation. When this separation is severe, the odontoid process could protrude into the foramen magnum and exert pressure on the spinal cord or impair blood flow through the vertebral arteries
- If flexion or awkward positioning is anticipated,
- Range of neck motion should always be evaluated preoperatively by asking the patient to demonstrate head movement or positioning.

Consider awake Fiber optic intubation.

Cardiovascular complications
- CAD.
- aortic regurgitation,
- conduction abnormalities
- Pericardial effusion.
- Pericarditis
- Tamponade
- conduction abnormalities

Pulmonary complications
- decreased thoracic mobility (restrictive lung disease),
- interstitial fibrosis,
- Pleural effusions.
- restrictive lung disease (thoracic restriction

Neurological complications
Vasculitis may lead to peripheral neuropathy
Renal complications
Renal dysfunction (worsened by NSAIDs
Gastroinstinal complications
- Chronic NSAID use (bleeding)
- Infectious: higher risk if on DMDs

Hashimoto's thyroiditis
causes
- autoimmune
- Medical/surgical treatment of hyperthyroid disease.

Preoperative preparation
Preoperative evaluation
- mild to moderate hypothyroidism is not an absolute contraindication to surgery.
- **Subclinical hypothyroidism** (elevated TSH with no clinical symptoms) is present in ~ 5% of patients (and 13% of elderly patients)
- Severe, symptomatic hypothyroidism can cause myxedema coma, pericardial effusion, and heart failure – if any of these are present, elective operations should be delayed until thyroid replacement has been initiated and is adequate.

Preoperative sedation
- Hypothyroid patients require less preoperative sedation and are prone to drug-induced respiratory depression,
- benadryl for sedation,
- metoclopramide for gastric-emptying (which is slowed).
- Euthyroid patients may receive their usual dose of thyroid medication on the morning of surgery .

Intraoperative management
Intubation may be complicated by a large tongue
Cardiac complications
- diminished cardiac output,
- blunted baroreceptor reflexes, and decreased intravascular volume, are at risk for severe hypotension.
- Induction may be best accomplished with ketamine
- . Consider pancuronium as a paralytic agent (chronoscopic effects).
- Do NOT give volatile anesthetics to hypothyroid patients, as they are at risk for severe myocardial depression.
- consider nitrous oxide plus intravenous agents (ex. benzodiazepines).
- There is no evidence that hypothyroid patients have reduced MAC requirements.

Monitoring
- Temperature control
- Cardiac output (i.e. avoiding congestive heart failure). In cases of refractory hypotension, one should always be cognizant of the possibility of acute adrenal failure.
- hypoglycemia,

- Anemia
- hyponatremia
- Hypothermia from a low basal metabolic rate.

Post operative recovery
Causes of delayed recovery from general anesthesia
- hypothermia,
- respiratory depression,
- slowed drug biotransformation
- hypothyroid patients often require prolonged mechanical ventilation
- opiates may need to be avoided to avoid respiratory depression
- ketorolac for postoperative analgesia.

Adrenal Disease
- **Adrenal Insufficiency**
- conditions often take steroid conditions often take steroids
- asthma
- COPD,
- autoimmune disease
- dermatologic,
- Placing them at risk for adrenal suppression that can last up to a year.
- Patient who has taken steroids for a month or more is usually replaced for a year there is some evidence

that these patients should be given physiologic doses of steroids in preparation for surgery.

Pheochromocytoma
- Rare cause of hypertension (~ 0.1%).
- 16% will have other, associated disorders.

Clinical picture
Initial diagnosis often made by the classic triad of tachycardia/palpitations, headache, and diaphoresis in the setting of hypertension.

Laboratory investigations
- VMA and metanephrines are the most specific tests.
- treatment
- Clonidine (which blocks sympathetic outflow) reduces blood pressure in essential hypertensives, but not in those with pheochromocytoma.

Preoperative preparation
- fluid resuscitated
- pre-established alpha-blockade (ex. phenoxybenzamine, prazosin)
- treat any arrhythmias if present (beta blockers).
- Note that alpha-blockers will enhance insulin release, decreasing blood glucose levels.

Intraoperative management
- Arterial line placement should proceed IV induction (avoid ketamine).

- Sevoflurane can be added prior to laryngoscopy in order to blunt the SNS response – DL should not occur until a surgical level of anesthesia has been obtained.
- fentanyl and IV lidocaine should be considered prior to intubation.
- Pancuronium should be avoided (because of its SNS stimulating effects). Nitroprusside should be available at induction.

Maintenance
- volatiles, which are ideal as they blunt the SNS.
- If MAC 1.5-2.0 does not adequately control blood pressure,
- nitroprusside infusion should probably be started.
- Note that when the veins are ligated, circulating catecholamine will drop rapidly, necessitating a reduction in volatile anesthesia as well as fluid resuscitation. Hyperglycemia (due to reduced alpha-induced insulin production) may ensue, thus glucose should be checked with regularity.
- Droperidol should be avoided, as it has been shown to cause a paradoxical hypertensive response (thought to be due to inhibition of norepinephrine reupdate.

Cushing's Disease
- Volume overloaded

- hypokalemic metabolic alkalosis due to the mineralocorticoid activity of excess glucocorticoids.
- Hypertension
- Diabetes
- Obesity
- Difficult airway

Obesity
Preoperative Considerations
- Overweight is defined as a BMI of 24 kg/m2,
- obesity as a BMI of 30,
- Morbid obesity as a BMI of 40.
- Cardiovascular complications of Obesity
- Hypertension
- Coronary artery diseases and cardiomegaly.
- Cardiac output has to increase 0.1 L/min/kg for adipose tissue (mostly accomplished through increased SV).
- VO2 is increased, as is CO2 production.

Pulmonary complications of obesity
- Obesity predisposes to obstructive sleep apnea syndrome
- Hypersensitivity to opiates as well as sedatives
- Obesity-hypoventilation syndrome (in 8% of patients
- Increases pulmonary blood pressure,
- Reduces FRC

- Expiratory reserve
- Decrease Vital capacity.

- FRC may fall below closing capacity, producing a baseline V/Q mismatch and hypoxemia.
- Hypercapnea is rare in obese patients
- hypoventilation syndrome (hypercapnea, cyanosis-induced polycythemia, respiratory failure, somnolence).
- Chest wall rigidity increases, further complicating mechanical ventilation.
- risk for aspiration (increased incidence of GERD and hiatal hernia),
- Many practitioners use a rapid sequence technique, and many authors recommend premedication with H2 blockers and metoclopramide.

Preoperative evaluation

Assess cardiopulmonary reserve.

Intraoperative management

- difficulties IV and intraarterial sites
- airway exam (limited mobility, shortened distance between mandible and sternal fat, lower FRC reduces time to desaturation).
- PEEP should be strongly considered intraoperatively.

Induction and Anesthesia

- Decreased FRC leads to more rapid changes in lung concentrations of volatile anesthetics.
- IV anesthetics are difficult to predict, as plasma volume is increased (decreases drug concentrations), but adipose tissue is not well-perfused

Anesthetic Dose requirement for obese patient
- Water soluble drugs as muscle relaxant adjusted according to lean body weight
- Fat soluble drugs as volatile anesthesia and narcotics Rarely need to dose based on more than 80 kg for females or 100 kg for males
- [Many drugs accumulate in adipose tissue, further complicating management, although obese patients may not be at increased risk for delayed emergenc.
- Obese patients have larger volumes of distribution for opiates and benzodiazepines (fat-soluble), thus some authors recommend larger loading doses and lower/less-frequent maintenance doses.
- Obese patients usually require 20–25% less local anesthetic (epidural fat, distended veins) and are at particular risk for respiratory compromise.

Post-Operative Considerations
- Respiratory failure is the major fear.
- The 45° modified sitting position unloads the diaphragm and improves ventilation/oxygenation.

- Consider routine post-operative supplemental oxygen for days, as PaO2 bottoms out at 2-3 days post-operatively.
- Incentive spirometry and early ambulation are helpful.
- Wound infection,
- deep venous thrombosis, and pulmonary embolism

Anesthetic considerations of Malnutrition

Elective surgery in patients who have lost 20% of their body weight should be postponed.
Enteral nutrition should be administered if possible, as outcomes are improved
TPN is only used when absolutely necessary
- fluid load,
- hyperchloremic metabolic acidosis
- excess CO_2 production
- Increased infection rates.

Diabetes
Complications of diabetes mellitus
<u>**Cardiovascular complications**</u>
- coronary artery disease
- peripheral vascular disease
- hypertension
- patients e on ACE-inhibitors (because of their renal sparing effects) or ARBs and may be at risk for severe hypotension at induction.

Central nervous system
- cerebrovascular strocke
- autonomic and sensory neuropathies [cardiovascular and GI effects]
- Diabetic patients may also be at increased risk for perioperative nerve injuries

Autonomic neuropathy
- Develops in ~ 1/3 of diabetics (50% of those with coexisting hypertension)
- Orthostatic hypotension,
- Reduced HR variability,
- Baseline tachycardia (decreased inhibitory input),
- Deep breathing,
- Prolonged QT interval
- Patients with the above symptomsmay be at increased risk for sudden death
- bradycardia non-responsive to atropine has been described in diabetic surgery patients.

joint stiffness
 TMJ and cervical joint stiffness (due to glycosylation of tissue proteins) should be assessed, as 30% of diabetics have difficult intubations.
Metabolic complications
- Diabetic ketoacidosis (DKA)
- **DKA** should be treated with fluid resuscitation, IV insulin (0.2 U/kg initially, 0.1 U/kg/hr after, goal is to decrease by 75–100 mg/dL or 10% per hour), and

K+ supplementation (some, but not all, authors recommend bicarbonate if pH is 7.2).

Hyperosmolar hyperglycemic non-ketotic coma
In elderly patients with thirst disturbances
Gastrointestinal complications
- Patients with autonomic symptoms (ex. gastroparesis)
- Risk for pulmonary aspiration.

Preoperative Evaluation
- coronary artery disease is the most common cause of perioperative mortality in diabetic patients,
- Chest pain (often absent), exercise tolerance, etc. should be sought.

Treatment of the Diabetic women

- Oral hypoglycemic doses are often held the morning of surgery, as patients are NPO and the risk of hypoglycemia is real.
- Metformin and sulfonylureas are often held for 24-48 hours before surgery. Metformin also carries with it the risk of metabolic acidosis.
- Insulin-dependent diabetics should receive insulin preoperatively, although there is no standardized dose – most commonly, ½ the daily dose is given as an intermediate acting agent after an IV is placed and glucose is checked.

Intraoperative Management

- IV lidocaine may help facilitate glycemic control [
- Insulin-dependent diabetics should have glucose monitored every 1-2 hours, with a goal of keeping glucose < 180.
- Do not rely on SQ or IM insulin intraoperatively, as these routes rely on adequate tissue perfusion.
- Consider starting a dedicated IV for D5W and IV insulin infusions (which could potentially interfere with other medications).

Cancer and women
Cancer common in women

- **Breast cancer** is the leading cancer for women in the US.
- **Lung cancer** is the second most common form of cancer
- **Colorectal cancer** is third among white women. The number 2 and 3 cancers are reversed among black and Asian/Pacific Island women.
- For all women, the fourth leading cancer is cancer of the **uterus**.

Possible causes of cancer

Environmental factors.

- Common environmental factors that contribute to cancer death include

- Tobacco (25–30%), diet and obesity (30–35%),
- Infections (15–20%),
- Radiation (both ionizing and non-ionizing, up to 10%),
- stress,
- lack of physical,
- environmental pollutants
- inherited genetics
- The remaining 5–10% are due.
- Lifestyle, economic and behavioral factors, and not merely pollution.

General symptoms

- unintentional weight loss,
- **fever**,
- being excessively tired,
- changes to the skin **Hodgkin disease**,
- **leukemias**, and **cancers of the liver** or **kidney** can cause a persistent **fever of unknown origin**

- most common places for metastases to occur are the **lungs**, **liver**, **brain**, and the bone

Cancer and anesthesia
Preoperative Evaluation

- Already systemic diseases ad hypertension , diabetes, ischemic heart diseases
- General complications of cancer,as anemia,loss of weight.
- Specific tumor complications,as electrolytes imbalance due to vomiting
- Metastesis in the lung, liver ,bone
- Chemotherapy and radiation systemic effects

preoperative Preparation
- Electrolyte abnormalities are common in patients with abdominal pain or vomiting, thus consider a preoperative chem.
- Blood products available + Ranger / rapid infuser.
- cefoxitin (do not give SQ heparin (5000 U) until AFTER the epidural, if placed).

Most common causes of death of cancer patients
 Sepsis, hemorrhage, and cardiovascular events
Induction/Airway: if the tumor is obstructive, consider RSI.
Intraoperative management
- Lines and Monitors:

- two large-bore IVs,
- Arterial line (frequent labs, esp. glucose).
- Central line.
- general +/- epidural (T6-8, inferior angle of scapula is approximately T7

Epidural anesthesia
- opiate-enhanced epidural is used, consider a lipophilic drug (ex.fentanyl),
- morphine will potentially spread rostrally,
- Potentially causing mental status changes and respiratory depression.
- Consider 0.5%bupivacaine intraoperatively, followed by 0.125% – 0.25% post-operatively.
- In patients for whom an epidural is not possible, consider ketamine at 0.2 mg/kg/hr after a 0.5 mg/kg bolus, as well asgabapentin 600-1200 mg PO.

Intraoperative Goals and Events:
- Placement of nasogastric tube (will be used post-operatively).
- WARM maintenance fluids at 6-10 cc/kg/hr.

Postoperative management
- Emergence: depends on fluid shifts and cardiopulmonary status. May remain intubated.
- ICU admission.
- Epidural-trained ward if epidural in place.

Cancer patients undergo chemotherapy before being subjected for surgery. Such patients pose some serious interactions and complications during the anaesthetic management.

Common complications associated with cancer chemotherapy agents

System toxicity	Chemotherapeutic agents
Cardiac toxicity	Busulphan, cisplatin, cyclophosphamide, daunorubucin, 5-fluorouracil
Pulmonarytoxicity	Methotrexate, bleomycin, busulphan, cyclophosphamide, cytarabine, carmustine
Renal toxicity	Methotrexate, L-asparginase, carboplatin, ifosfamide, mitomycin-C
Hepatic toxicity	Actinomycin D, methotrexate, androgens, L-asparginase, busulphan, cisplatinum, azathiopine
CNS toxicity	Methotrexate, cisplatin, interferon, hydroxyurea, procarbazine, vincristine
SIADH secretion	Cyclophosphamide, vincristine

The most common toxicities to chemotherapeutic agents
- Cardiac,
- Pulmonary,
- Hematologic,
- Bone marrow
- Gastrointestinal effects.
- Coagulopathies, thrombocytopenia,
- anemia with ulceration and bleeding of the gastrointestinal tract

Cardiovascular effects and complications following chemotherapy

Anthracyclines; i.e. doxorubicin (adriamycin), daunorubicin, and epirubicinare the commonest agents implicated in the development of cardiac toxicity after cancer chemotherapy.

Three types depending on their appearance in relation to timing of therapy,

Anthracycline agents may impair myocardial contractility.

Risk factors for development of anthracycline cardiotoxicity:

1. high dose radiation to the mediastinum
2. concurrent cyclophosphamide therapy
3. extremes of age,
4. prior ischaemic heart disease,
5. hypertension,
6. valvular heart disease and liver diseases.
7. cumulative dose in the range of 300-450 mg/m2 is about 1-10%, while doses higher than this invites a risk of>30%.

Pathogenesis ofanthracycline cardiotoxicity:
- The anthracycline antibiotics react with cytochrome P-450 reductase in the presence of reduced nicotinamide adenine dinucleotide phosphateto form semiquinone radical intermediates, which in turn can react with oxygen to form superoxide anion radicals.
- These can generate both hydrogen peroxide and hydroxylradicals, which are highly destructive to cells thus causing myofibrillarlysis, cytoplasmic vacuolization, and degeneration of nuclei and mitochondria in the myocytes. Severe myocyte damage results in decreased myocardial contractility and CHF.

Investigations for the detection of anthracycline cardiotoxicity:
- radionucleide angio-cardiography. The
- left ventricular ejection fraction (LVEF). A decrease in LVEF to less than 45% is considered to indicate anthracycline-induced cardiotoxicity. 2-Dechocardiography is a non-invasive method of cardiac valuation.
- Diastolic dysfunction on echocardiogram may represent an earlier manifestation of anthracycline toxicity.
- The newer noninvasive methods to know the actual myocardial damage are by using imaging with monoclonal indium–111–antimyosin antibodies.
- These antibodies bind to the exposed myosin in the necrosed myocardial cells.

- A diffuse uptake on imaging indicates a generalised process such as anthracycline cardiomyopathy; a focal uptake will suggest local pathology such as myocardial infarct.**mitoxantrone** at a total dose of more than 140 mg/m2 can suffer congestive heart failure
- anthracycline-induced cardiomyopathy.

Dysrhythmias:
- **dysrhythmias** unrelated to the cumulative dose
- dysrhythmias may occur hours or even days after administration.
- Commonly observed dysrhythmias include supraventricular tachycardia, complete heart blocks, and ventricular tachycardia.

- Doxorubicin may prolong the QT interval.
- anthracyclines may enhance the myocardial depressive effect of anesthetics even in patients with normal resting cardiac function.

cyclophosphamide causes myocardial tissue injury
A **cyclophosphamide** dose range of more than 120mg.kg−1 over 2 days can result in severe congestive heart failure and haemorrhagic myocarditis, pericarditis, and necrosis.
busulfan oral daily dosage may suffer endocardial fibrosis, with signs and symptoms of constrictive cardiomyopathy.

Patients with preexisting cardiac disease receiving interferon in conventional doses may have exacerbations of their underlying illness.

mitomycin for extended periods of time and dosages has been shown to produce myocardial damage.

paclitaxel, with cisplatinum, may also produce ventricular tachycardia

The preoperative and anesthetic assessment

- 2D-echocardiogram or nuclear medicine studies.
- Measurement of the left ventricular ejection fraction and detection of regional and global myocardial dysfunction. Where congestive failure is discovered, the physician will have to treat it preoperatively.

Types of cardiac toxicty
Acute and Subacute cardiotoxicity:

- It can occur immediately after a single dose or a course of anthracycline therapy.
- Acute toxicity commonly (40%) takes the form of ECG changes such as nonspecific ST-T changes, decreased QRS voltage, and QT prolongation
- Decreased R wave amplitude has been thought by some to signal development of chronic cardiomyopathy later, though it is not proved.
- Sinus tachycardiais the most common rhythm disturbance but avariety of arrhythmias, including ventricular, supraventricular, and junctional tachycardia, have been reported.
- Atrioventricular and bundle-branch block have.

- These changes occur at all dose intervals and except for decreased QRS voltage, resolve 1 to 2 months after cessation of the therapy.
- Sudden death may also occur, due to ventricular fibrillation.
- Rare cases of subacute cardiotoxicity resulting in acute failure of the left ventricle, pericarditis or a fatal pericarditis-myocarditis syndrome, particularly in children, have been reported.
- If these patients recover they should not receive further treatment with anthracyclines
- In elderly patients with preexisting heart disease, congestive heart failure can occur, which is generally transient and responds to normal medical management.

Chronic or late cardiotoxicity:
- Chronic cardiotoxicity after anthracyclines classically takes the form of cardiomyopathy. CXR review may reveal cardiomegaly.
- ECG changes occur with these agents and includenon-specific ST-and T-wave changes, prematureatrial and ventricular contractions, sinus tachycardia and low-voltage QRS complexes.
- Anthracycline cardiotoxicity is a cumulative dose related phenomenon.
- The incidence of congestive heart failure secondary to anthracycline induced cardiotoxicity increases with dose.

- The rapid increasein incidence of CHF after a dose of 550 mg/m2 has made it a popular empiric-limiting dose for doxorubicin-induced cardiotoxicity.

Late onset cardiotoxicity:
- occultventricular dysfunction, heart failure and arrhythmias occurring in previously asymptomatic patients more than a year after anthracycline therapy.
- Doxorubicin can cause subclinical myocardial injury during pre-adolescent years and this in later years retards appropriate growth of the myocardium during growth spurt.

<u>Anesthetic management:-</u>
- Invasive monitoring techniques hinges on thorough pre-operative assessment.
- Invasive arterial blood pressure recordings and apulmonary artery catheterization may be necessary if significant myocardial impairment is present.
- Anthracycline treated patients under anaesthesia can develop acute intraoperative left ventricular failure refractory to β- adrenergic receptor agonists.
- Amrinone and sulmazole are the new class of cardiotonics with inotropic drugs useful in such conditions.

B) **Pulmonary effects and complications of cancer chemotherapy**
- 75% to 90% of pulmonary complications are secondary to infection.
- The cancer patient can suffer infectious complications secondary to chemotherapy (e.g., Bleomycin), thoracic radiation, and multiple pulmonary resections.
- respiratory failure in cancer patients requiring assisted mechanical ventilation is associated with a 75% mortality rate
- Pulmonary infiltrates seen on a routine chest radiograph is extensive; there are many causes for such infiltrates.
- busulfan, cyclophosphamide, paclitaxel, etc, can lead to pulmonary complications. Bleomycin, an antitumour agent, producing lung damage.

Bleomycin pulmonary toxicity produced by have been described:
- About 0-40% patients are reported to develop pulmonary toxicity
- 11-30% patients will have non-lethal pulmonary fibrosis and the mortality associated with bleomycin toxicity will range from 2-10%.

The risk factors for bleomycin pulmonary toxicity
- Old age
- Accumulative dose >400-450 U

- Poor pulmonary reserves
- Radiotherapy
- Uremia, higher inspired oxygen concentrations
- Concomitantly administered other anticancer drugs

Mechanisms of pulmonary toxicity:

- the threshold dose level for the development of pulmonary disease is in the range of 400 to 450mg,
- Fatal pulmonary fibrosis has been reported with doses as low as 50mg.
- The mechanism of pulmonary toxicity associated with the use of bleomycin, is probably due to direct cytotoxicity and in patients receiving bleomycin, type I pneumocytes are replaced by type II pneumocytes.
- Continued exposure to bleomycin prevents reversion of type II to type I pneumocytes and further leads to meta-plasia of the type II cells to cuboidal epithelium.
- Further exposure prevents effective repair and fibrosblasts and macrophages migrate into the interstitium and the alveoli.

- Another mechanism for bleomycin toxicity involves the production of superoxide and other free radical moieties, Cleave nuclear DNA.

- The production of these highly oxidizing radicals might be increased by the inspiration of fortified concentrations of oxygen.

Pathology of chemotherapy pulmonary toxicity

- Dose dependent interstitial pneumonitis progressing to chronic fibrosis
- An acute hypersensitivity pneumonitis with peripheral eraleosinophilia resembling eosinophilic pneumonia.
- An acute chest pain syndrome.
- A bronchitis obliterans with organising pneumonia.
- Pulmonary veno-occlusive disease.
- Progressive interstitial pneumonitis and fibrosis is the most common pattern of bleomycin lung injury.

Clinical picture of pulmonary toxicty

- Symptoms generally occur between 4 to 10 weeks after bleomycin therapy,
- 20% patients with radiographic and histological features of bleomycin toxicity may be present without any clinical symptoms.

Clinical presentation:
- The lesions seen frequently are in the lower lobes and sub pleural areas and chest X-ray shows bilateral basal and peri-hilar infiltrates with fibrosis.
- The first signs and symptoms of toxicity are fever, cough, dyspnoea and bibasilar rhonchi and rales, which may progress to exertional dyspnoea with mild X-ray changes and a normal resting PaO2or a severe form of hypoxia at rest.
- The earliest detection of pulmonary fibrosis may be achieved through the serial evaluation of pulmonary function.
- Sequential measurement of carbon monoxide diffusion capacity (DLCO) may indicate the presence of occult pulmonary changes.
- Arterial hypoxemia is commonly found and spirometry reveals decreased lung volumes compatible with restrictive lung disease.
- Regression or amelioration of the toxic pulmonary pathology may occur with immediate cessation of therapy. Steroid therapy has been found to be effective in some cases.
- Noncardiogenic pulmonary edema, chronic pneumonitis and fibrosis, and hypersensitivity pneumonitis.

Anesthetic management of pulmonary toxicty:

- Importance to the anaesthesio logist is the debate about the amount of oxygen to be administered to a patient coming up for surgery after being given bleomycin.
- Perioperative oxygen restriction is not necessary
- Perioperative fluid balance including transfusions as a significant predictor of postoperative pulmonary morbidity.
- The duration of surgery and post-chemotherapy forced vital capacity are significant predictive factors of procedure related pulmonary morbidity.
- On the basis of available data it seems prudent to reduce the concentration of inspired oxygen to the lowest level to maintain SpO2 > 90%.
- Use of intraoperative PEEP to enhance oxygenation
- Fluid balance is another important factor in predicting pulmonary morbidityin-patients receiving bleomycin.
- Conservative fluid management is important; use of colloids is beneficial as compared to crystalloid.

Intraoperative monitoring

Arterial blood gas analysis should be performed by an indwelling arterial cannula or intermittent sampling.

Post operative care

Postoperative use of rigorous physiotherapy to treat ventilation-perfusion abnormalities may

Effects of cancer chemotherapy agents on hepato-renal, and CNS system

Renal complications:-

- Cisplatinum, a commonly used anticancer drug has been found to produce toxic effects like nephrotoxicity, myelosuppression, neuropathy in stocking and glove distribution, auditory and visual impairment.

- The dose-limiting factor for single agent use, however, is nephrotoxicity. 30% of patients receiving cisplatinum will develop nephrotoxicity, especially if the hydration is not properly controlled.

Mechanism of renal complications of chemothrapy

- It causes coagulation necrosis of proximal and distal renal tubular epithelial cells and in the collecting ducts leading to are duction in the renal blood flow and glomerular filtration rate (GFR).
- Cisplatinum leads to wasting of magnesium and potassium. A single dose of 2mg/kg or 50-75mg/m2 will produce nephrotoxicity in 25-30% of patients.
- The newer analogues of cisplatinum, such as carboplatinum and oxaloplatinum are less nephrotoxic with equal efficacy in controlling the malignancy.
- Methotrexate causes the acute nephrotoxicity as a result of its intratubular precipitation

Acute renal failure

- **Acute renal failure** can result within 24 hours of administration of a single dose of cisplatinum.
- Use of normal saline is particularly beneficial as high chloride concentrations in the tubules inhibit the hydrolysis of cisplatinum.
- The renal toxicity may be accentuated if the patient receives aminoglycosides concomitantly.

CNS complications:-

- Vinca alkaloids were the first anticancer drugs found to have neurotoxiceffects.
- Vincristine is probably the only drug whose dose limiting toxicityis neurotoxicity.
- It can affect the central, peripheral or the autonomic nervous systems. Peripheral neuropathies present as peripheral paresthesias with depression of deep tendon reflexes.
- The paresthesias progress proximally with therapy. Motor dysfunction and gait disorders can occur.
- Vincristine, vinblastine, procarbazine, cisplatinum
- all can cause a toxic neuropathy with paresthesia, loss of deep tendon reflexes and muscle weakness.
- Autonomic neuropathy with orthostatic hypotension is a rare concomitant of neoplasia
- Cranial nerve effects may manifest as opthalmoplegia and facial palsy
- Autonomic neuropathy can present asorthostatic hypotension, erectile dysfunction, constipation, difficulty in micturition, bladder atony, et
- **Cisplatinum**, along with its effects on the kidney also affects the nervous system. 50% patients receiving cisplatinum will display neurotoxicity

depending on dose and treatment duration. It generally takes the form of paresthesias.

- Continued treatment will lead to loss of deep tendon reflexes, vibration sense and sensory ataxia.

Regional anesthesia and neuropathy

- regional anaesthesia is concerned, one should be aware that in a considerable percentage of patients a sub-clinical, unrecognized neuropathy may be present in patients with previous cisplatinum chemotherapy.
- Recently, a diffuse brachial plexopathy after interscalene blockade has been reported in a patient receiving cisplatinum chemotherapy.
- Thus, if regional anaesthesia is contemplated, a detailed pre-operative neurological examination .

Hepatic complications:-

- Hepatocellular dysfunction is manifested as raised serum enzymes,
- fatty infiltration of liver and cholestasis, due to direct toxic effect of the drug or it's metabolite.
- L-asparginase and cytarabine are most commonly implicated agents in hepatocellular dysfunction.
- A decreased synthetic function with low proteins and coagulation abnormalities may be seen.Ascites, painful hepatomegaly, and encephalopathy may result after administration of cytarabine, cyclophosphamide, mitomycin, etc.

Haematological complications:-

- Bone marrow function in cancer patients may be disturbed by primary bone marrow disorders (e.g., leukemia), bony metastases (e.g., from breast cancer), as well as myelosuppressive chemotherapy.
- The production of any or all blood elements may be impaired. There is dysfunctional coagulation. The PT and PTT are shortened. There is increase in factor I, V, VIII, IX, XI and FDP.
- There is reduced survival of the platelets and the decreased antithrombin III activity.
- Some investigators have maintained a minimal level of 50,000 platelets per microliter in the intraoperative and postoperative period. Correction of other coagulation disturbances is important before undertaking surgical intervention in the thrombocytopenic patient.
- Close cooperation among the surgeon, anaesthesiologist, and hematologist is required for optimal management and maximal safety.
- Myelo-suppression caused by all the chemotherapeutic agents is partially or completely reversible within 1 to 6 weeks of termination of therapy.

Syndrome of inappropriate antidiuretic hormone secretion (SIADH):-

- Another metabolic abnormality in patients with cancer like lung, pancreas-adeno-carcinoma, duodenum, thymoma, mesothelioma, leukaemia, hodgkin, reticulum cell sarcoma, is SIADH, which occurs in 1% to2% of cancer patients.
- Some drugs, such as vasopressin, carbamazepine, oxytocin, vincristine, vinblastine, cyclophosphamide, phenothizianes, tricyclic antidepressant agents, narcotics, and monoamine oxidase inhibitors, can also induce SIADH.

Steroid administration:

- The oncology patient often has a history of exogenous glucocorticoid administration as part of a chemotherapy regimen.
- The physician at the time of pre-operative evaluation has to decide on the use and the amount of stress steroid coverage.
- The patient who has received ≥2 weeks of glucocorticoids within the past year is considered at risk for adrenal suppression.
- However, many of these patients are capable of a normal stress response. The corticotrophin (ACTH) stimulation test is the definitive test to identify adrenal suppression.

Tumorlysis syndrome:-

- Chemotherapy induces rapid tumor cell lysis in patients with a large malignant cell burden over an exquisitely sensitive tumor
- This classically occurs in patients with Burkitt's lymphoma, non-Hodgkin's lymphomas, acute lymphoblastic and nonlymphoblastic leukemias, and chronic myelogenous leukemia.
- In addition, it may also occur continuously in patients with lymphomas and leukemia following treatment with chemotherapy, radiation, glucocorticoids, tamoxifen, or interferon. The clinical mani-festations of this syndrome are related to the metabolic abnormalities.
- In those patients with suspected tumor lysis syndrome or for those patients who receive chemotherapeutic agents likely to induce the syndrome, prevention is the mainstay of treatment.
- To prevent the development of acute renal failure, patients who are to undergo treatment for malignancies should receive vigorous intravenous hydration, often with diuretics or renal doses of dopamine to ensure adequate urine output

Chemotherapy and wound healing:-

- The outcome of surgical procedures may be affected by the wound-healing impairment caused by antineoplastic agents used to treat the underlying tumor. The neutropenia that accompanies some chemotherapy within 7 to 10 days of administration can interfere with the early phases of wound healing..

- The effects of chemotherapy directly on wound healing depend on doseand the timing of drug administration relative to creation of the wound.
- A high incidence of wound complications has been reported in women undergoing mastectomy after receiving preoperative chemotherapy and radiation. Bleomycin has not been associated with increased wound complications.

Osteoporosis

Osteoporosis is a disease that weakens bones, increasing the risk of sudden and unexpected fractures.

Osteoporosis results in an increased loss of bone mass and strength. The disease often progresses without any symptoms or pain

steoporosis is a systemic skeletal disorder characterized by compromised bone strength, low bone mass, and disruption of bone architecture, predisposing to an increased risk of fracture.

The World Health Organization (WHO) defines osteoporosis as having a bone mineral density (BMD) at the hip or lumbar spine greater than 2.5 standard deviations below the young normal adult reference population.

High risk factors for osteoporosis in women

- activity level

- How much calcium
- family history
- history of taking certain medications
- Lifestyle habits, such as whether smoke or how much alcohol consume
- The onset of menopau
- **Prevention**

Calcium supplements, loss of weight, exercises, stop smoking

Causes of osteoporosis in women

Menopause

- Estrogen is important for maintaining bone density in women.

- When estrogen drops after menopause, bone loss speeds up.

- This can happen with natural menopause or an early surgical menopause if you have your ovaries removed.

- During the first five to 10 years after menopause, women can lose about 2.5% of bone density each year. That means they can lose as much as 25% of their bone density during that time.

- Accelerated bone loss after menopause is a major osteoporosis in women. For women, having the strongest bones possible *before you enter menopause* is the best protection against debilitating fractures.

Drugs cause osteoporosis

1. Steroid-induced osteoporosis (SIOP) arises due to use of glucocorticoids – analogous to Cushing's syndrome and involving mainly the axial skeleton. The synthetic glucocorticoid prescription drug prednisone is a main candidate after prolonged intake. Some professional guidelines recommend prophylaxis in patients who take the equivalent of more than 30 mg hydrocortisone (7.5 mg of prednisolone), especially when this is in excess of three months. Alternate day use may not prevent this complication.
2. Barbiturates, phenytoin and some other enzyme-inducing antiepileptic – these probably accelerate the metabolism of vitamin D.

3. L-Thyroxin over-replacement may contribute to osteoporosis, in a similar fashion as thyrotoxicosis does. This can be relevant in subclinical hypothyroidism.

4. drugs induce hypogonadism, for example aromatase inhibitors used in breast cancer, methotrexate and other antimetabolite drugs, depot progesterone andgonadotropin-releasing hormone agonists.

5. Anticoagulants – long-term use of heparin is associated with a decrease in bone density, and warfarin (and related coumarins) have been linked with an increased risk in osteoporotic fracture in long-term use.

6. Proton pump inhibitors – these drugs inhibit the production of stomach acid; this is thought to interfere with calcium absorption. Chronic phosphate binding may also occur with aluminum-containing antacids.

7. Thiazolidinediones (used for diabetes) – rosiglitazone and possibly pioglitazone, inhibitors of PPARγ, have been linked with an increased risk of osteoporosis and fracture.

8. Chronic lithium therapy has been associated with osteoporosis.

Certain diseases are at increased risk of osteoporosis

- rheumatoid arthritis
- ankylosing spondylitis,

- systemic lupus erythematosus
- polyarticular juvenile idiopathic arthritis ,
- Systemic diseases such as amyloidosis and sarcoidosis can also lead to osteoporosis.
- Renal insufficiency can lead to renal osteodystrophy.
- Hematologic disorders linked to osteoporosis are multiple myeloma,and other monoclonal gammopathies,
- lymphoma and leukemia, mastocytosis,
- hemophilia, sickle-cell disease and thalassemia
-

Anesthesia and osteoprosis
- Women are exposed to anesthesia when fractures occur.
- Vertebral fractures are the most common osteoporotic fracture in postmenopausal women. It is estimated that there are 550,000 to 700,000 osteoporotic vertebral compression fractures (VCFs) annually, which account for ~27% of all osteoporotic fractures in both men and women

Anesthetic precution for osteoporosis
- Gentel intubation for cervical vertebrae protection ,fibroptic intubation may be needed to avoid excessive extension of the neck
- Care for transportation, to avoid any fractures and dislocations.

- Care for positioning
- Stress dose of cortisol if indicated if the patient is with regular administration.

DEPRESSION

- One of the common women's diseases is depression.
- Depression is the most common psychiatric disorder, affecting 10–20% of the population, and is characterized by sadness and pessimism
- The highest prevalence of depression among women than men is due to higher risk of first onset.
- Gender difference first emerges in puberty,
- Changes in sex hormones (pregnancy, menopause, use of oral contraceptives, and use of hormone replacement therapy)
- Effects of biological vulnerabilities and environmental provoking experiences.
- Anesthesia and surgery react direct and indirect with the antipsychotic drugs.
- The anesthesiologist must be aware of potential interactions with anesthetic agents.
- There are profound effects on the central and peripheral neurotransmitter and ionic mechanisms when Psychotropic drugs often given in combination with each other or with other non-psychiatric drugs generally exert.

The risk of interaction between anesthesia and antidepression drugs depends on:

- The extent of surgery
- The patient's physical state
- Anesthesia, the direct and indirect effects of psychotropics,
- Risk of withdrawal symptoms
- Risk of psychiatric recurrence and relapse.

Types of antidepressent drugs

- Tricyclic antidepressants (TCA),
- Selective serotonin re-uptake inhibitors,
- Atypical agents and monoamine oxidase inhibitors (MAOIs).
- Atypical antidepressants include venlafaxine and mirtazapine.
- Both these drugs should be continued throughout the perioperative period.
- About 70–80% of the patients respond to antidepressant medications.

DISCONTINUATION SYNDROME
Abrupt cessation of antidepressants is associated with the risk of developing withdrawal symptoms,
symptoms

- nausea,
- abdominal pain
- diarrhoea,

- sleep disturbance,
- somatic symptoms (sweating, lethargy and headache)
- Affective symptoms (low mood, anxiety and irritability).

These reactions start abruptly within a few days of stopping the antidepressant, are short lived (a few days to 3 weeks) and end if the antidepressant is reintroduce

selective serotonin reuptake inhibitors (SSRIs)
- Drugs in this group include amitriptyline, imipramine, desipramine, doxepin, nortriptyline and others.
- Desipramine and nortriptyline are used as tricyclic antidepressant as they are less-sedating.

TCAs
- Inhibit synaptic reuptake of norepinephrine and serotonin.
- They also affect other neurochemical systems including histaminergic and cholinergic systems.

Side-effects
- Postural hypotension
- Cardiac dysrhythmias
- Urinary retention
- Dry mouth
- Blurred vision and sedation.

ECG

- T wave changes, widening of the QRS complex and prolongation of QT interval, bundle branch block or other conduction abnormalities, or PVCs.
- Ventricular arrhythmias and refractory hypotension may occur at higher doses.

Anesthesia and TCA

Increase anesthetic requirements, increased availability of neurotransmitters in the central nervous system .

anticholinergics

- Atropine cross the blood–brain barriermay cause postoperative confusion.
- Exaggerated blood pressure responses following administration of indirect acting
- Vasopressors such as ephedrine due to increased availability of norepinephrine at the post-synaptic nervous

Pancuronium, ketamine, meperidine and epinephrine containing solutions should be avoided.

1. Exaggerated response to both indirect acting vasopressors
2. Sympathetic stimulation
3. If hypotension occurs and vasopressors are needed, direct acting drugs such as phenylephrine are recommended. The dose should probably be decreased to minimize the likelihood of an exaggerated hypertensive response.

4. During anesthesia and surgery, it is important to avoid stimulating the sympathetic nervous system.

Potentiating the cardiac depressant effects of anesthetic agents

Chronic therapy with tricyclic antidepressant drugs depletes cardiac catecholamine.

Selective serotonin reuptake inhibitors (SSRIs

Mechanism of action:
- SSRIs block reuptake of serotonin at the pre-synaptic membranes,
- With relatively little effect on adrenergic, cholinergic, histaminergic or other neurochemical systems.

Side-effects
- They are associated with few side-effects.
- Examples include fluoxetine, paroxetine and sertraline.
- Headache, agitation and insomnia.
- Among SSRIs, fluoxetine is a potent inhibitor of certain hepatic cytochrome P-450 enzymes.
- This drug may increase the plasma concentration of drugs that depend upon hepatic metabolism for clearance, such as warfarin, theophylline, phenytoin and benzodiazepines.
- Antidysarrhythmic drugs are also metabolized by this enzyme system, and fluoxetine inhibition of the

enzyme system may result in potentiation of their effects.

Anesthetic precaution with SSRIs
SSRIs should be continued throughout the perioperative period to prevent discontinuation syndrome.
Avoid the use of pethidine, tramadol, pentazocine and dextromethorphan.

Serotonin syndrome
Serotonin syndrome is a potentially life-threatening adverse drug reaction that results from increased serotonin levels in the brain stem and spinal cord. A large number of drugs have been associated with the serotonin syndrome. These include SSRI, MAOI, TCAs, pethidine, tramadol and dextromethorphan.

Clinical features
- Behaviour (agitation and confusion),
- Increased motor activity and autonomic instability (hyperthermia, tachycardia, labile blood pressure and diarrhea.
- Seizures, rhabdomyolysis, renal failure, arrhythmias, coma and death may

MAOIs
MAOIs, tranylcypromine and phenelzine, and the selective and reversible MAOIs, moclobemide,

MECHANISM OF ACTION
- Inhibition of the metabolic breakdown of norepinephrine and serotonin by the MAO enzyme.

- The level of norepinephrine and serotonin is increased at the receptor site. All MAOIs are eliminated by hepatic metabolism

Interactions between MAOIs and anaesthetic drugs
There are two distinct types of reaction that can occur between MAOIs and opioids.
Type I (excitatory)
Reactions occur in patients given pethidine and dextromethorphan, both of which inhibit serotonin reuptake.
CLINICAL PICTURE
Serotonin syndrome
- pethidine and dextromethorphan remain contraindicated.
- Other opioids like morphine, fentanyl, alfentanyl and remifentanyl can all be used safely.

Type II (depressive) reaction
- It is very rare, is thought to be due to MAO inhibition of hepatic enzymes resulting in enhanced effects of all opioids.
- It is reversed by naloxone.

Indirect acting sympathomimetics
- It precipitates potentially fatal hypertensive crisis and are absolutely contraindicated with any MAOIs.
- Direct acting sympathomimetics (adrenaline, noradrenaline and phenylephrine) may have an enhanced effect due to receptor hypersensitivity
- Dosages should be titrated.

- Phenelzine decreases plasma cholinesterase concentration and prolongs the action of suxamethonium.
- Pancuronium should be avoided as it releases stored noradrenaline.
- MAOIs may cause a reduction in the hepatic metabolism of barbiturates, resulting in reduction of the dose requirement of thiopentone.
- Propofol and etomidate can be used safely. Ketamine should be avoided as it causes sympathetic stimulation.
- Local anesthetics containing adrenaline should be used with caution.
- Benzodiazepines, inhalational anesthetic agents, anticholinergic drugs and non-steroidal anti-inflammatory drugs can be used safely in patients taking MAOIs.

Anesthesia for a patient on MAOIs
- MAOI is to be stopped, the doses should be reduced gradually and with regular psychiatric review.
- Cancellation of surgery should be avoided and the treatment restarted as soon as possible post-operatively.
- In a patient on MAOIs or in the emergency situation, benzodiazepine premedication can be given and sympathetic stimulation should be avoided. Adequate hydration of the patient should be ensured.

- Hypotension should be treated initially with intravenous fluids and then with cautious doses of phenylephrine.
- Pethidine and indirect acting sympathomimetics are absolutely contraindicated

References

1. *Barnett SR, Morin RJ, Kiely DK, Gagnon M, Azhar G, Knight EL, Nelson JC, Lipsitz LA. Effects of age and gender on autonomic control of blood pressure dynamics. Hypertension 33: 1195–1200, 1999.*

2. *Bar-or O, Shephard RJ, Allen C. Cardiac output of 10- to 13-year-old boys and girls during submaximal exercise. J Appl Physiol 30: 219–223, 1971*

3. *Bevegård S, Shepherd JT. Regulation of the circulation during exercise in man. Physiol Rev 47: 178–213, 1967*

4. *Buckey JC Jr, Lane LD, Levine BD, Watenpaugh DE, Wright SJ, Moore WE, Gaffney FA, Blomqvist CG. Orthostatic intolerance after spaceflight. J Appl Physiol 81: 7–18, 1996*

31. Foley JF. Complications of chemotherapy agents. In: Foley J, Vose J, Armitage JA, editors. Current Therapy in Cancer. 2nd edn. Philadelphia: W. B.Saunders; 1999. pp. 485–491.

32. Burrows FA, Hickey PR, Colan S. Perioperative complications in patients with anthracycline chemotherapeutic agents. Can Anaesth Soc J. 1985;32:149–157. [PubMed]

33. Lahtinen R, Kuikka J, Nousianinen T, et al. Cardiotoxicity of epirubicin and doxorubicin: A double-blind randomized study. Eur J Haematol. 1991;46:301–305. [PubMed]

34. Lekakis J, Vassilopoulos N, Psichoyiou H, et al. Doxorubicin cardiotoxicity detected by indium 111 myosin-specific imaging. Eur J Nucl Med. 1991;18:225–226. [PubMed]

35. Weesner KM, Bledsoe M, Chauvenet A, et al. Exercise echocardiography in the detection of anthracycline

cardiotoxicity. Cancer. 1991;68:435–438. [PubMed]

36.Lewkow LM, Hooker JL, Movahed A. Cardiac complications of intensive dose mitoxantrone and cyclophosphamide with autologous bone marrow transplantation in metastatic breast cancer. Int J Cardiol.1992;34:273–276. [PubMed]

37.Solley GO, Maldonado JE, Gleich GJ, et al. Endomyocardiopathy with eosinophilia. Mayo Clin Proc.1976;51:697–708. [PubMed]

38. Drzewoski J, Kasznicki J. Cardiotoxicity of antineoplastic drugs. Acta

39.Haematol Pol. 1992;23:79–86.[PubMed]

40. Verweij J. Mitomycins. Cancer Chemother Biol Response Modif. 1996;6:48–56. [PubMed]

41.Huettemann E, Junker T, Chatzinikolaou KP, et al. The influence of anthracycline therapy on cardiac function during anesthesia. Anesth Analg. 2004;98:941–947. [PubMed]

42. Steinherz LJ, Steinherz PG, Tan CT, et al. Cardiac toxicity 4 to 20 years after completing

anthracycline therapy. JAMA. 1991;266:1672–1677. [PubMed]

43. Burrows FA, Hickey PR, Colan S. Perioperative complications in patients with anthracycline chemotherapeutic agents. Can Anaesth Soc J. 1985;32:149–157. [PubMed]

44. Cortes JE, Pazdur R. Docetaxel. J Clin Oncol. 1995;13:2643–2655. [PubMed]

45. Steinberg JS, Cohen AJ, Wasserman AG, Cohen P, Ross AM. Acute arrhythmogenecity of doxorubicin administration. Cancer. 1987;60:1213–8. [PubMed]

46. Bristow MR, Billingham ME, Mason JW, Daniels JR. Clinical spectrum of anthracycline antibiotic cardiotoxicity. Cancer Treat Rep. 1978;62:873–79. [PubMed]

47. 18. Lefor AT. Perioperative management of the patient with cancer. Chest. 1999;115:165S–171S. [PubMed]

48. 19. Praga C, Beretta G, Vigo PL, Pollini C, Bonadonna G, Canetta R, et al. Adriamycin cardiotoxicity: A survey of 1273

patients. Cancer Treat Rep. 1979;63:827–834. [PubMed]

49. Von Hoff DD, Layward MW, Basa P, Davis HL, Jr, Von Hoff AL, Rozencweig M, et al. Risk factors for doxorubicin–induced congestive heart failure. Ann Intern Med. 1979;91:710–717. [PubMed]

50.Shan K, Lincoff AM, Young JB. Anthracycline-induced cardiotoxicity. Ann Intern Med. 1996;125:47–58.[PubMed]

51.Steinherz LJ, Steinherz PG, Tan CT, Heller G, Murphy ML. Cardiac toxicity 4 to 20 years after completing anthracycline therapy. JAMA. 1991;266:1672–77. [PubMed]

52. Lipshultz SE, Colan SD, Gelber RD, Perez Atayde AR, Sallan SE, Sanders SP. Late cardiac effects of doxorubicin therapy for acute lymphoblastic leukemia in childhood. N Engl J Med. 1991;324:808–15. [PubMed]

53.Ganz WI, Sridhar KS, Ganz SS, Chakko S, Serafini A. Review of tests for monitoring Doxorubicin-induced

Cardiomyopathy. Oncology. 1996;53:461–470. [PubMed]

54. Varon J. Acute respiratory distress syndrome in the postoperative cancer patient. The Cancer Bulletin.1995;47:38–42.

55. Dumont P, Wh JM, Hentz JG, et al. Respiratory complications after surgical treatment of esophageal cancer: A study of 309 patients according to the type of resection. Eur J Cardiothorac Surg. 1995;9:539–543. [PubMed]

56. Epner De, White F, Krasnoff M, et al. Outcome of mechanical ventilation for adults with hematologic malignancy. J Invest Med. 1996;44:254–260. [PubMed]

57. Randle CJ, Jr, Frankel LR, Amylon MD. Identifying early predictors of mortality in pediatric patients with acute leukemia and pneumonia. Chest. 1996;109:457–461. [PubMed]

58. Lombara CM, Churg A, Winokur S. Pulmonary veno-occlusive disease following therapy for malignant neoplasms. Chest. 1987;92:871–876. [PubMed]

59.Meysman M, Schoors DF, Reynaert H, et al. Respiratory failure with diffuse patchy lung infiltrates: An unusual presentation of squamous cell carcinoma. Thorax. 194(49):1271–1272. [PMC free article] [PubMed]

60. Williams DM, Krick JA, Remington JS. Pulmonary infection in the compromised host: Oncol Biol Part I. Am Rev Respir Dis. 1976;114:359–394. [PubMed]

61.Waid-Jones M, Coursin DB. Perioperative considerations for patients treated with bleomycin. Chest.1991;99:993–99. [PubMed]

62. Rosenow EC, 111, Myers JL, Swensen SJ, et al. Drug-induced pulmonary disease: An update. Chest.1992;102:239–250. [PubMed]

63. Goldiner PL, Schweizer O. The hazards of anesthesia and surgery in Bleomycin-treated patients. Seminars in Oncology. 1979;6:121–124. [PubMed]

64.Goldiner PL, Carlon GC, Cvitkovic E, Schweizer O, Howland W. Factors influencing postoperative morbidity and mortality in patients treated with bleomycin. Britsh Medical

Journal. 1978;1:1664–1668. [PMC free article][PubMed]

65. LaMantia KR, Glick JH, Marshall BE. Supplemental oxygen does not cause respiratory failure in Bleomycin-treated surgical patients. Anesthesiology. 1984;60:65–67. [PubMed]

66. Donat SM, Levy DA. Bleomycin associated pulmonary toxicity: is perioperative oxygen restriction necessary?The Journal of Urology. 1998;160:1347–52. [PubMed]

67. Madias NE, Harrinton JT. Platinum nephrotoxicity. Am J Med. 1978;65:307–14. [PubMed]

68. Fjeldberg P, Sorensen J, Helkjaer PE. The long term effects of cisplatin on renal function. Cancer.1986;58:2214–17. [PubMed]

69. El-Badawi MG, Abdalla MA, Bahakim HM, Fadel RA. Nephrotoxicity of low-dose methotrexate in guinea pigs: an ultrastructural study. Nephron. 1996;73:462–466. [PubMed]

70. Weiss HD, Walker MD, Wiernik PH. Neurotoxicity of commonly used antineoplastic agents. NEJM.1974;291:75–81. [PubMed]

71. Kedar A, Cohen ME, Freeman AI. Peripheral neuropathy as a complication of cis-Dichlorodiammine-platinum treatment: a case report. Cancer treatment reports. 1978;62:819–821. [PubMed]

72. Siemsen JK, Meister L. Bronchogenic carcinoma associated with severe orthostatic hypotension. Ann Int Med. 1963;58:669–676. [PubMed]

73. Huettemann, Egbert Sakka, Samir G. Anaesthesia and anti-cancer chemotherapeutic drugs. Anaesthesia and medical disease. Current Opinion in Anaesthesiology. 2005;18:307–314. [PubMed]

74. Heyman MR. Cancer and therapy-related hematologic abnormalities. In: Lefor AT, editor. Surgical problems affecting the patient with cancer. Philadelphia PA: Lippincott-Raven; 1996. pp. 373–392.

75. Anderson RJ, Chung HM, Kluge R, et al. Hyponatremia: A prospective analysis of its epidemiologyand the pathogenetic role of vasopressin. Ann Intern Med. 1985;102:164–168. [PubMed]

76. Fleming DR, Doukas MA. Acute tumor lysis syndrome in hematologic mahgnancies. Leuk Lymphoma.1992;8:315–318. [PubMed]

77. Jones DP, Mahmoud H, chesney RW. Tumor lysis syndrome: Pathogenesis and management. Pediatr NephroI.1995;9:206–212. [PubMed]

78. Van der Hoven B, Thunnissen PL, Sizoo W. Tumour lysis syndrome in haematological malignancies. Neth J Med. 1992;40:31–35. [PubMed]

79. Scha¨ffer MR, Barbul A. Chemotherapy and wound healing. In: Lefor AT, editor. Surgical problems affecting the patient with cancer. Philadelphia, PA: Lippincott-Raven; 1996. pp. 305–320.

80. Mathes DD, Bogdonoff DL. Preoperative evaluation of the cancer patient. In: Lefor AT,

editor. Surgical problems affecting the patient with cancer. Philadelphia, PA: Lippincott-Raven; 1996. pp. 273–304.

81. Klein DS, Wilds PR. Pulmonary toxicity of antineoplastic agents: anaesthetic and postoperative implications.Can Anaesth Soc J. 1983;30:399–405. [PubMed]

82. Zsigmond EK, Robins G. The effect of a series of anticancer drugs on plasma cholinesterase activity. Can Anaesth Soc J. 1972;19:75–82. [PubMed]

83. Frenia ML, Long KS. Methotrezate and NSAID interactions. Ann Pharmacother. 1992;26:234–237.[PubMed]

84. Walsh, SJ, LM. Autoimmune Diseases: A Leading Cause of Death among Young and Middle-Aged Women in the United States. American Journal of Public Health. 2000;90:1463-1465

85. U.S. Department of Health and Human Services. Office on Women's Health. Women's Health Issues: An Overview. Fact sheet. May 2000.

86. Society for Women's Health Research and the National Women's Health Resource Center, Inc. Autoimmune Diseases in Women.2002.

87. National Women's Health Information Center. U.S. Department of Health and Human Services, Office on Women's Health. WomensHealth.gov/faq/lupus.pdf

www.ingramcontent.com/pod-product-compliance
Lightning Source LLC
Chambersburg PA
CBHW060403190526
45169CB00002B/724